中华传统经典养生术

（汉英对照）

(Chinese-English) Traditional and Classical Chinese Health Cultivation

Chief Producer Li Jie	总策划 李 洁
Chief Compilers Li Jie Xu Feng Xiao Bin Zhao Xiaoting	总主编 李 洁 许 峰 肖 斌 赵晓霆
Chief Translator Han Chouping	总主译 韩丑萍
English Language Reviewer Lawrence Lau	英译主审 劳伦斯·刘

天柱导引功

Tian Zhu Dao Yin Gong

编著 肖 斌
Compiler   Xiao Bin

翻译 韩丑萍
Translator   Han Chouping

上海科学技术出版社
Shanghai Scientific & Technical Publishers

图书在版编目（CIP）数据

天柱导引功：汉英对照 / 肖斌编著；韩丑萍译.
—上海：上海科学技术出版社，2015.5
（中华传统经典养生术）
ISBN 978-7-5478-2559-4

Ⅰ.①天… Ⅱ.①肖… ②韩… Ⅲ.①气功–健身运
动–基本知识–汉、英 Ⅳ.①R214

中国版本图书馆CIP数据核字（2015）第042961号

天柱导引功

编著 肖 斌

上海世纪出版股份有限公司
上海科学技术出版社 出版
（上海钦州南路71号 邮政编码200235）
上海世纪出版股份有限公司发行中心发行
200001 上海福建中路193号 www.ewen.co
上海中华商务联合印刷有限公司印刷
开本 787 × 1092 1/16 印张 7.75
字数：80千字
2015年5月第1版 2015年5月第1次印刷
ISBN 978-7-5478-2559-4/R·877
定价：68.00元

顾问委员会

编纂委员会

Compilation Committee Members

总策划

李 洁

Chief Producer

Li Jie

总主编

李 洁　许 峰　肖 斌　赵晓霆

Chief Compilers

Li Jie　Xu Feng　Xiao Bin　Zhao Xiaoting

副总主编

孙 磊　陈昌乐　倪青根

Vice Chief Compilers

Sun Lei　Chen Changle　Ni Qinggen

总主译

韩丑萍

Chief Translator

Han Chouping

副主译

赵海磊

Vice Chief Translator

Zhao Hailei

项目资助

Acknowledgement

· 上海市新闻出版专项扶持资金项目

· 上海市中医药三年行动计划（2015—2018年）"基于〈中华气功史陈列馆〉科普教育基地为核心的〈中医气功文化平台〉建设"（项目编号：ZY3-WHJS-1-1010）

· Shanghai Press and Publication of special support funds program

· The Three-Year Action Plan for Chinese Medicine in Shanghai (2015–2018) on Construction of Qigong Cultural Platform in the Museum of Chinese Qigong History (Program No: ZY3–WHJS–1–1010)

序

Foreword

欣闻上海市气功研究所编写的《中华传统经典养生术》丛书即将出版,这是中华原创医学文明传播的一件盛事,特致贺忱。

中华传统养生术源远流长,其中导引术更是重要的组成部分,它先于针、灸、药、医而形成,是中华民族最早用以防治疾病、养生保健的重要方法之一。现存早期文献《庄子》《吕氏春秋》《黄帝内经》以及考古发现《引书》《导引图》中均有关于养生导引及其具体方法的记载。此后绵绵数千年的历史长河中,中华养生导引术不断丰富、发展与创新,在自我实践中形成千门万法,在去伪存真中完善理论体系。20世纪后叶,古之导引术又以现代"气功"的面目再次席卷中华大地,并享誉海内外。时至今天,中华导引术仍然以其"人天合一"的整体观思想与丰富多姿的养生导引方法独立于世界自然医药之林,滋润着人类身心世界。事实表明,中华导引术已经形成为一门博大精深的学术体系。它所研究的是人之物质基础(精)与自组织能力(神)相互关系的规律,是关于"人"——这个地球上最复杂系统达到和谐与协调的一门学问。

我和上海市气功研究所相识逾30年,该所自20世纪70年代的中医研究所开始,气功与导引就是关注、研究的重点领域;80年代中期更名气功研究所后,更是全力着眼于现代气功的研究与中华导引术的弘扬。《中华传统经典养生术》是上海市气功研究所多年来所教授养生导引术、气功功法的汇编与总结,对于帮助学习、普及推广现代导引术具有较好的价值。希望此丛书的出版,能够进一步带动当前养生导引术在海内外的健康发展,推动中华优秀文化走向世界各地。

是以为序。

林中鹏

2015年3月

It is with great pleasure that I learn the *Traditional and Classical Chinese Health Cultivation* series compiled by the Shanghai Qigong Research Institute will be published soon. This means a lot to the spread of Chinese medical civilization.

Traditional Chinese health cultivation has a long-standing and well-established history. As an important part of health cultivation practice, Dao Yin exercise was used for disease prevention and treatment as well as life cultivation before acupuncture, moxibustion and herbal medicine. The recordings of *Dao Yin* and its specific exercise methods can be traced back to the *Zhuangzi, Lü Shi Chun Qiu* (The Annals of Lü Buwei), *Huang Di Nei Jing* (the Yellow Emperor's Inner Classic) and archaeologically unearthed books such as *Yin Shu* (a book on Dao Yin) and *Dao Yin Tu* (Dao Yin Diagram). After this, the thousands of years have witnessed the enrichment, progress and innovation of Chinese *Dao Yin* practice, coupled with emergence of numerous methods and perfection of its theoretical system. In late 20th century, the ancient *Dao Yin* exercise became exceptionally popular across China in the form of 'qigong'. Today, Chinese *Dao Yin* exercise remains flourish with its holistic 'Man-Nature Unity' idea and various exercise methods that benefit both body and mind. Facts show that there is a profound academic system behind Chinese *Dao Yin* exercise. This system studies the interactions between material foundation (essence) and self-organization ability (mind). In other words, it studies the way to achieve harmony and coordination of human being—the most complex system on earth.

I've established a friendship with the Shanghai Qigong Research Institute for 30 years. Ever since its founding in 1970s as a Research Institute of Chinese Medicine, qigong and *Dao Yin* have always been the research priorities of the Institute. The focuses on qigong and *Dao Yin* have been more highlighted in 1980s when the Institute was renamed as a Qigong Research Institute. I firmly believe that the

Traditional and Classical Chinese Health Cultivation series are of great significance in popularizing modern *Dao Yin* exercise. I sincerely wish the book series can further promote *Dao Yin* exercise at home and abroad and spread excellent Chinese culture.

For this, I wrote this forward.

Lin Zhongpeng

March 2015

前　言

Preface

气 以 臻 道

农历乙未早春，正是上海市气功研究所创建三十周年之际，恰逢气功学术发展枯木迎春之季。在此，我们谨向海内外气功学界发出倡言——构建现代气功"气以臻道"的学术思想。

所谓"气以臻道"，首先是指气功学术发展必须树立一个大方向，即中华传统文化精神的最高目标——"道"；其次是指通过对"气"的感性体验与理性认知，使生命更趋向"道"，与"道"合一。道者，规律、目标也；气者，方法、途径也；臻者，趋向、完善也。气－道共同构成"气以臻道"学术思想内核。其中气为实、主行，是具体之指；道为虚、主理，是抽象之喻。气因道而展，道由气而实；气以道归，道以气显；气借道而实际指归，道假气而理性论证。气功学术发展必须气、道并重，互印互证，理行一贯。两者既各尽其责、各擅其能，又有主从之别。"道"因标指形上本体而为万法归宗之源；"气"每描述形下万法而成法法生灭之流。"道"经思维抽象提炼，揭示规律、规则之理性思辨；"气"常直叙主观感觉，表述体会、觉受的感性认识。道－气，一主一从，一虚一实，构成中华气功学术思想的本质内涵。

"气以臻道"学术思想之主体是"道"，是指向真理之道路，是学术文化人文精神的体现，也是先人用身心去实践生命运化规律的心得体验，古人称为"内证之学"。"道"的外延旁及"功"和"术"，可以包括各种神秘现象、气功现象、特异现象，古人称为"神通法术"。当今，现代科学研究介入传统气功学术是时代进步的表现，它为我们观察生命奥秘打开了一个全新的视角。透过唯象的研究，重新激发起人类对生命的思考与敬重，重新挖掘出科技文明下的人文精神，而非单纯地将生命物质化，这才是现代科学介入传统气功的人文价值所在。

　　有鉴于此，我们倡议构建现代气功研究之"气以臻道"学术思想，让中华传统文化与现代科学携起手来，揭示生命真谛，回归大道本源。

上海市气功研究所

2015年春

Advocacy for *Qi-Dao Harmony* in Modern Qigong Practice

The year 2015 is a Chinese new year of yin wood sheep (*Yi Wei* in Chinese). Wood, in Chinese culture on five elements (*Wu Xing*), is connected to the season of spring. The year 2015 also marks the 30th anniversary of the founding of Shanghai Qigong Research Institute. With a strong belief that the spring of 2015 will bring new hope to qigong study, we hereby advocate the concept of 'Qi-*Dao Harmony*' for its academic advance.

The term *Qi-Dao Harmony* has two underlying implications. First, it implies that *dao* is the ultimate goal of traditional Chinese culture and the general orientation for academic qigong advance. Second, it implies that our lives shall combine into one with the *dao* through perception and understanding of qi. In summary, this term means to achieve and perfect *dao* through qi exercise. The 'qi' here is weighted and refers to practice. The '*dao*' here is unweighted and refers to principles. Without *dao*, qi cannot extend; without qi, *dao* cannot become weighted. Qi finds its origin in *dao* and *dao* manifests itself in qi. Qi returns to *dao* eventually and *dao* supports qi theoretically. It's essential for people in academic qigong field to pay equal attention to qi and *dao*. The two have a principal-subordinate relationship. The metaphysical *dao* is the origin of all methods. The physical qi is the practice of all methods. *Dao* is about the abstract thinking and reveals the laws and rules. Qi is about the subjective feelings and tells experience and perception. Qi and *dao* constitute the essence of academic idea in Chinese qigong.

Let's get a deeper look into the concept of *Qi-Dao Harmony*. Also known as the 'learning of internal evidence', *dao* is the way to truth. It contains humanistic spirit and physical and mental experience of our ancestors. *Dao* extends to exercise (*gong*) and a variety of magic arts including mysterious, qigong and extrasensory phenomena. Today, modern scientific qigong research offers a new insight into the mysteries of life. The phenomenological research rekindles our reflection and respect towards life and enables us to re-discover humanism from modern civilization greatly impacted by science and technology. This is the real value of scientific research on traditional qigong in this materialized world.

To this end, we advocate the academic concept of '*Qi-Dao Harmony*' in modern qigong research. We believe the combination of traditional Chinese culture and modern science can help us to reveal the truth of life and return to the origin of the great *dao*.

Shanghai Qigong Research Institute
Spring 2015

编写说明

Words from the Compilers

中华传统养生术根植于中国传统哲学、中医学和养生学，是人体自我身心锻炼的有效方法。

随着倡导"主动健康"概念日益深入人心，具有调身、调息、调心功能的中华传统养生术，以其传统的养修理论、独特的身心效果蜚声海内外，引起世人的广泛关注。但近期国内外少见中国传统养生术的书籍出版，尤其没有成套、成系列的经典养生类作品问世，更缺乏英汉对照的专业著作。

上海中医药大学上海市气功研究所研究人员在前期研究工作基础上，精选中华传统经典养生术共八种，从历史源流、功法理论、特色要领、图解动作、分解说明与具体运用几方面进行中文编纂，由上海中医药大学中医英语专业人员进行翻译。并邀请专家进行中文审稿，邀请美国友三中医药大学 Lawrence Lau 先生审定英文翻译。

本套丛书详细地将八种中华经典养生术以图文并茂、视频摄像的形式记录下来，配以光盘，非常方便学习与传播，尤其便于海外养生爱好者以英语来学习。

本套丛书编纂过程中，得到上海市中医药三年行动计划（2015—2018年）"基于〈中华气功史陈列馆〉科普教育基地为核心的〈中医气功文化平台〉建设"（项目编号：ZY3-WHJS-1-1010）资助。

编者

Traditional Chinese health cultivation includes a variety of body-mind exercises, which are deeply rooted in ancient Chinese philosophy and medicine.

Today, the concept of 'health initiative (an ability to achieve physical, mental and social well-being)' has become well recognized.

Traditional Chinese health cultivation exercises are attracting worldwide attention because of their unique effects in regulating the breathing, body and mind. However, there are few books in this regard, especially the classical book series. There are even fewer bilingual Chinese-English versions of these books.

Based on their previous studies, research staff at the Shanghai Qigong Research Institute compiled eight traditional and classical health cultivation exercise methods, covering their history, theoretical foundation, characteristics and key principles, illustrated movements and application. Then these contents have been translated by professional interpreters at Shanghai University of Traditional Chinese Medicine. The Chinese version was reviewed by an expert team. The English version was reviewed by Dr. Lawrence Lau at the Yo San University of Traditional Chinese Medicine.

In addition to illustrations and videos are also available for readers, especially overseas health cultivation fans to learn.

This books series have been funded by the Three-Year Action Plan for Chinese Medicine in Shanghai (2015–2018) on Construction of Qigong Cultural Platform in the Museum of Chinese Qigong History (Program No: ZY3–WHJS–1–1010).

Compilers

目 录

Table of Contents

天 柱 导 引 功 · *Tian Zhu Dao Yin Gong*

History

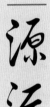

天柱即是人体脊柱,因其支撑人体全身,取其擎天一柱之意,故名天柱。天柱导引功是传统养生导引功法之一,它主要是通过脊柱的伸展、屈曲、旋转、侧曲等不同的导引动作来疏通经脉,平衡阴阳,调和脏腑气血以达到祛病健身养生的目的。它的功法内容可以追溯到秦汉时期的导引术,在西汉马王堆出图的导引图中可以找到它的源头,它是在继承中国古代导引术的基础上,吸取了各家之长,把人体多种"导引"的精华与练丹田相结合,把人体动静与人体神意相结合,把练功与保健相结合而成,它是由著名的气功医家董妙成老师继承和传授的,并经气功专家如马济人、林厚省、沈鹤年等协助进一步完善,成为上海市气功研究所传统养生功法之一。

Tian Zhu literally means heavenly pillar. In this text, it refers to the human spine, since the spine supports our body frame in an upright position. As a traditional *Dao Yin* exercise, Tian *Zhu Dao Yin Gong* aims to unblock meridians, balance yin and yang, harmonize qi and blood of zang-fu organs and achieve health through stretching, flexion, rotation and lateral bending of the spine. Its origin can be traced back to *Dao Yin* gymnastics in Qin (221–207BC) and Han (206BC–AD220) dynasties. A case in point is the *Dao Yin Tu* (Dao Yin Diagram) of the Western Han dynasty (206BC-AD 24) unearthed from the Han Dynasty Tomb Mawangdui. *Tian Zhu Dao Yin Gong* combines ancient Daoyin techniques with Dantian concentration, body movements with mental focus, and qigong practice with health cultivation. As one of the classical qigong exercises in Shanghai Qigong Research Institute, *Tian Zhu Dao Yin Gong* was inherited by qigong master Dong Miao-cheng and further developed by qigong experts including Ma Ji-ren, Lin Hou-sheng and Shen He-nian.

根据现代医学研究，脊柱为人体的中轴骨骼，是身体的支柱，有负重、减震、保护和运动等功能。脊柱由26块脊椎骨合成，即24块椎骨（颈椎7块、胸椎12块、腰椎5块）、骶骨1块、尾骨1块，由于骶骨系由5块，尾骨由4块组成，故正常脊柱也可以说由33块组成。这样众多的脊椎骨，由于周围有坚强的韧带相连系，能维持相对稳定，又因彼此之间有椎骨间关节相连，具有相当程度的活动度。在脊柱椎体与棘突之间为椎管，内藏脊髓，脊髓两旁发出许多成对的神经（称为脊神经）分布到全身皮肤、肌肉和内脏器官。脊髓是周围神经与脑之间的通路，也是许多简单反射活动的低级中枢。脊柱外伤时，常合并脊髓损伤。严重的脊髓损伤可引起下肢瘫痪、大小便失禁等。人体自主神经是调节、控制各脏腑功能的神经，分为交感与副交感神经，与脊髓有密切关系，人体在正常情况下，功能相反的交感和副交感神经处于相互平衡制约中。在这两个神经系统中，当一方起正作用时，另一方则起负作用，很好的平衡协调和控制身体的生理活动，这便是自主神经的功能。

In modern medicine, spine is axial skeleton and backbone of the body. It supports our body frame in an upright position, acts as shock absorbers from load-bearing, protects the spinal cord and associated nerves and allows for movement. The spine consists of 26 vertebrae — 24 vertebrae (7 cervical vertebrae, 12 thoracic vertebrae, and 5 lumbar vertebrae), 1 sacral bone and 1 tail bone. Since there are 5 sacral bones and 4 tail bones, the normal spine is composed of 33 bones. Stability of these vertebrae is maintained by strong ligaments. Facet joints with each vertebra allow the flexibility and movement of these vertebrae. The spinal canal is enclosed within the vertebral foramina. It is the space in vertebrae through which the spinal cord passes. Pairs of spinal nerves (one on each side of the vertebral column) are distributed over the skin, muscles and internal organs. The spinal cord is the main pathway for information connecting the brain and peripheral nervous system. It is also the hub of many simple reflections. Severe spinal cord injury resulting from trauma can cause paralysis or incontinence. The autonomic nervous system has two branches: the parasympathetic nervous system (PSNS), and the sympathetic nervous system (SNS). Normally, PSNS and SNS have "opposite" actions where one system activates a physiological response and the other inhibits it.

本功法通过脊柱的锻炼，能改善脊柱和脊髓的气血循环，使脊柱筋骨强健，蕴含"一柱擎天"而生生不息之意，并能调节神经功能，对很多慢性病有很好的防治作用。

Through exercise of the spine, *Tian Zhu Dao Yin Gong* can improve the qi and blood circulation of the spine and spinal cord, strengthen the spine, regulate nerve function and prevent or treat chronic conditions. *Tian Zhu Dao Yin* implies to use one pillar to prop up the sky and generate endless vitality.

人体的脊柱特别是脊髓在传统养生和传统医学中称为督脉，是人体最重要的经脉，属于奇经八脉之一，为阳脉之总督，称为阳脉之海。督脉阳气通畅，则全身百脉皆通，脏腑功能调达，就可以达到身健而百病消、心宁而寿绵长的养生目标。

In traditional health cultivation and Chinese medicine, human spine is in the pathway of one of the eight extraordinary meridians — Du meridian. Du meridian governs all yang meridians and is known as the sea of yang meridians. Unblocked yang qi of Du meridian secures smooth qi and blood flow in other meridians and normal functioning of zang-fu organs. As a result, one can achieve health and longevity.

天 柱 导 引 功 · *Tian Zhu Dao Yin Gong*

Theoretical Foundation

理论基础

经络与气功

Meridians and Qigong

经络学说是中医学理论的重要组成部分,它贯穿在生理、病理、诊断、治疗、预防等各个方面,从基础理论到临床各科,都占有重要的位置。它同样也是气功学的基础。在《黄帝内经》中对经络及其有关问题,作了大量的论述,尤其是《灵枢》,按照《黄帝内经》所述,经络是气血在机体内运行的特殊通路,它们"内属于腑脏,外络于肢节"(《灵枢·海论》)。

As an important part of Chinese medicine, meridian theory is extensively used in physiology, pathology, diagnosis, treatment and prevention and plays a key role in fundamental theory and clinical subspecialties. It is also the foundation of qigong. The *Huang Di Nei Jing*[1] (Yellow Emperor's Internal Classic), especially the *Ling Shu* (Spiritual Pivot) recorded detailed discussions on meridians (special pathways for qi and blood circulation), 'Internally, they connect with the zang-fu organs; externally, they connect with the surface of the body' (*Ling Shu Hai Lun*).

经络系统分为经脉与络脉,循行于机体深处的直行主干称作经,分布于肌表的分支称作络。经有正经十二条、奇经八条。根据阴阳学说的演绎,把十二经分为手足三阳经和手

---

1. An ancient Chinese medical text that has been treated as the fundamental doctrinal source for Chinese medicine for more than two millennia, the work is composed of two texts — Su Wen (Basic Questions) and Ling Shu (Spiritual Pivot).

足三阴经两大类。经络的作用主要有：沟通表里上下，联系脏腑器官；通行气血，濡养脏腑组织；感应传导；调节人体各部分机体，使之保持相对平衡。传统气功学认为在经络中运行的经气，是元气中最活跃的部分，也是被称为内气的一部分，通过练功可以被人感知。传统气功学中还认为经络更是练精化气、练气化神的渠道。经气运行的特点是："流行不止，环周不休""如环之无端，莫知其纪，终而复始"（《素问·举痛论》）。

Meridian system includes meridians and collaterals. Meridians travel in deeper area longitudinally. Collaterals are branches distributed over the surface of the body. There are twelve regular meridians and eight extraordinary meridians. Based on yin-yang theory, the twelve regular meridians are divided into three yang-meridians of hand and foot and three-yin meridians of hand and foot. Major functions of meridians are to connect interior (zang-fu organs) with exterior (surface of the body), circulate qi and blood to nurture zang-fu organs and balance the body. Traditional Qigong theory holds that meridian qi is the most active part of yuan-primordial qi, also known as internal qi that can be perceived through qigong practice. Qigong theory also holds that meridians are pathways to transform essence into qi and transform qi into spirit. 'The flow of meridian qi does not stop and it circulates without break.' (*Su Wen Ju Tong Lun*)

气功与经络的关系中，与奇经八脉更为密切。因为奇经八脉有调节十二正经的作用，正如李时珍在《奇经八脉考》中说："盖正经犹夫沟渠，奇经犹夫湖泽，正经之脉隆盛，则溢于奇经。"反之，当沟渠流量小时，也需湖泽之水给予渗灌。所以奇经八脉对十二经起着调盈济虚的作用。而奇经八脉中更以督、任两脉与气功息息相关。因为"督脉起于会阴后，为阳脉之总督，故曰阳脉之海。任脉起于会阴，循腹而行于身之前，为阴脉之承任，故曰阴脉之海"（《奇经八脉考》）。按督脉所以称它为"总督诸阳"或"阳脉之海"，因为它循行于背部正中，其脉气多次与十二正经中的手、足三阳的全部六条阳经相交会，最集中的位置是大椎穴，手足三阳经都在这里左右相会，其次带脉出于第二腰椎绕腰一圈，阳维脉与督脉也交会在风府、哑门，这样督脉就起着统率的作用了。任脉所以称"阴脉之海"，因为它循行于胸腹正中，并在中极穴与足三阴经交会，在天突穴、廉泉穴与阴维脉交会，在阴交穴与冲脉交会，同时足三阴经上接手三阴经于胸腹，这样任脉就可以沟通手、足三阴经的全部六条阴经。

Qigong is more associated with the eight extraordinary meridians, since they can regulate the twelve regular meridians. Li Shi-zhen[1] states in the *Qi Jing Ba Mai Kao* (Textual Research on Eight Extraordinary Meridians), 'The twelve regular meridians are like irrigation canals and ditches, whereas the eight extraordinary meridians are like lakes and reservoirs. When the canals and ditches are full to the brim, the eight extraordinary meridians can take the overflow'. In other words, when the twelve regular meridians are deficient, they can supplement and support. Of the eight extraordinary meridians, Du and Ren meridians are especially related to Qigong, 'Du meridian originates from the lower abdomen and governs all yang meridians, and it is therefore called sea of yang meridians. Ren meridian originates from the lower abdomen and travels along the front midline, and it is therefore called sea of yin meridians (*Qi Jing Ba Mai Kao*)'. The word *Du* means to govern (yang). Du meridian (the sea of yang meridians) travels along the spine and crosses with three-yang meridians of hand and

---

1. Li Shi-zhen (1518–1593): One of the greatest Chinese physicians, herbalists and acupuncturists in history. His major contribution to clinical medicine was his 27-year work, which is found in his book Compendium of Materia Medica (*Ben Cao Gang Mu*).

foot (six yang meridians), particularly at Dazhui[1] (DU 14). The Dai meridian goes round the waist like a belt. Du meridian crosses with Yangwei meridian at Fengfu[2] (DU 16) and Yamen[3] (DU 15). On the nape, Ren meridian (sea of yin meridians) travels along the midline of the chest and abdomen. It crosses with three foot-yin meridians at Zhongji[4] (Ren 3), with Yinwei meridian at Tiantu (Ren 22) and Lianquan (Ren 23) and with Chong meridian at Yinjiao[5] (Ren 7). The three foot-yin meridians connect with three hand-yin meridians at the chest and abdomen. As a result, Ren meridian connects with all six yin meridians of hand and foot.

李时珍在《奇经八脉考》对此更直接指出："任督两脉，乃身之子午也，乃丹家阳火阴符升降之道，坎水离火交媾之乡。"也就是说任督两脉是内气（经气）循环升降之隧道。传统气功中还认为任督两脉督领百脉，如俞琰注《参同契》云："人身血气，往来循环，昼夜不停，医书有任、督两脉，人能通此两脉，则百脉皆通，自然周身流转，无有停壅之患，而长生久视之道断在此矣。"

Li Shi-zhen also states in the *Qi Jing Ba Mai Kao* that, 'Du meridian and Ren meridian are like midnight and midday, they are the pathway for yang ascending and yin descending and foundation for coordination between kidney water and heart fire'. Traditional qigong theory also holds Du and Ren meridians

---

1. An acupuncture point located in the depression below the spinous process of C7.
2. An acupuncture point located on the nape, 1 cun directly above the midpoint of the posterior hairline, directly below the external occipital protuberance, in the depression between the trapezius muscles of both sides.
3. An acupuncture point located on the nape, 1.5 cun directly above the midpoint of the posterior hairline, below the 1st cervical vertebra.
4. An acupuncture point located on the lower abdomen and on the anterior midline, 1 cun below the centre of the umbilicus.
5. An acupuncture point located on the lower abdomen and on the anterior midline, 1 cun below the centre of the umbilicus.

are the spearheads of the other meridians. The *Zhou Yi Can Tong Qi* (Token for the Agreement of the Three According to the Book of Changes) by Yu Yan records, 'Blood and qi within the human body flow without break. There are Du and Ren meridians in medical books. If Du and Ren meridians are unblocked, all the other meridians are unobstructed. As a result, one can achieve health and longevity'.

天 柱 导 引 功 · *Tian Zhu Dao Yin Gong*

Characteristics and Essential Principles

特色与要领

功 法 特 色

Characteristics of *Tian Zhu Dao Yin Gong*

　　本功法是在继承了中国古代导引术的基础上，吸取了各家之长，把人体多种"导引"的精华与练丹田相结合，把人体动静与人的神意相结合，把练功与保健相结合而成的传统导引类功法，它具有以下特色。

Tian Zhu Dao Yin Gong combines *Dao Yin* exercise with Dantian concentration, body movements with mental intent and qigong practice with health cultivation. Its characteristics are summarized as follows:

伸
Stretching

　　本功法通过脊柱的伸展、旋转、侧弯以及屈曲等不同的摆动，使脊柱及其周围的组织得到充分的锻炼，伸筋拔骨，能疏通以督脉为主的经脉，温通阳气，增强气血循环，还能带动四肢及内脏的气血运行，在松静自然与形神合一中达到祛病健身的目标。

Through stretching, rotation, lateral bending and flexion of the spine, this exercise can work on the spine and its surrounding tissue, stretch the tendons and bones and fully unblock Du meridian. Furthermore, it can warm yang qi, enhance the circulation of qi and blood in four limbs and zang-fu organs, obtain mind-body unity in relaxation and tranquility and promote health.

松
Relaxation

在练功中要做到形松体松，还要求做到心松意松，要在身心两方面避免紧张，消除紧张，使全身处于放松舒适的状态之中，有利于进入气功状态。在本功法中通过不同的功法来放松，有通过脊柱的拧转、拔伸、弯曲等来放松的，有用拍打经络关节来放松的，也有通过拉伸大筋而先紧后松的，通过习练能使全身完全放松。

A full relaxation of body and mind is essential for qigong practice. This exercise involves a couple of relaxation methods. These include spinal rotation, stretching and bending, tapping the meridians and stretching the large tendons.

静
Tranquility

本功法在练习时强调静心凝神，集中注意力，克服心中纷起的杂念，使身心处于一种安定祥和的状态，并且让注意力能集中在功法动作与呼吸上，让呼吸、意识与动作密切结合，使三调相互融合，慢慢进入一种通达自在的练功境界。所谓心定则气和，气和则血顺，血顺则精足而神旺，精足神旺者，内气充盈，疾病自然消除。

This exercise stresses a tranquil mind, concentration and free of distracting thoughts. It's essential to focus the mental intent on body movements and breathing. Only by integrating breathing, mental consciousness and body movements, can one enter a carefree qigong state. This is what we call 'a tranquil mind leads to even breathing, an even breathing leads to smooth blood circulation, a smooth blood circulation leads to essence and energy, and abundant internal qi can remove pathogenic factors out of the body'.

功 法 要 领
Essential principles of *Tian Zhu Dao Yin Gong*

松紧结合、伸筋拔骨
Combine intensity with relaxation and stretch tendons and bones

　　松静自然，即体松心静，是指在气功锻炼的具体操作过程中，都必须强调在以身体放松和心理放松的条件下进行，这是气功锻炼的基本原则。因为每个人的身体条件，气脉关节等情况都不相同，所以本功法中要求松紧结合，有松有紧，通过拉伸大筋、拧转脊柱、站桩等做到伸筋拔骨，通利关节，先紧后松，以达到使身心完全放松的目的。

A relaxed body and a tranquil mind are essential for qigong practice. Since body constitution, qi, vessels and joints vary greatly from person to person, *Tian Zhu Dao Yin* Gong combines intense exercise with relaxation methods. Stretching the tendons, rotating the spine and *Zhan Zhuang* can benefit joints and fully relax the body and mind.

动静结合、刚柔相济

Combine motion with stillness and integrate hardness with softness

本功法属导引动功，在练动功时，要求动中有静，外形运动而神意安静，意念集中，此即所谓动中寓静。在本功法中也有特定的站桩功法，站桩属于静功，通过站功可极大的增强经络气血的运行，即所谓静中含动。故动与静的有机结合，既有益于外在的形体运动，又有益于内气的聚集与运行，能够有效地提高练功效果。本功法有刚有柔，要求寓柔于刚，寓刚于柔，刚而不僵，柔而不散，刚柔相济而蕴含内劲，气意鼓荡而真气充实。

As a dynamic *Dao Yin* exercise, *Tian Zhu Dao Yin* Gong combines active body movements with inner tranquilization (mental focus). Static *Zhan Zhuang* in this exercise can enhance the circulation of qi and blood. Integrated motion and stillness can benefit physical movements as well as flow of internal qi, and thus improve the exercise effect. In addition, movements of *Tian Zhu Dao Yin Gong* are soft but not loosened, hard but not rigid. They are perfect combination of softness in hardness and hardness in softness, containing genuine qi and internal strengthen.

姿势准确、持之以恒

Keep accurate postures and be perseverant

准确活泼是要求在本功中进行肢体动作、自我按摩、自我拍击时，它的姿势一定要正确，动作要合乎规范，这样才能收到更好的效果。要求对动作的起落、高低、轻重、虚实都要分辨清楚；对举动、部位、手法、次数、神态、用意、呼吸，也都要记清和掌握。练功养生需要一个较长期的过程，所以要求习练者要有毅力和恒心，坚持不懈，持之以恒，以达到祛病健身、益智开慧、延年益寿的功效。

Body movements, self-massage and tapping are required to be lively but accurate. Accurate postures and movements are associated with better exercise results. To do this, you need to be clear about the lifting, dropping, high, low, gentle, heavy, weighted or unweighted movements. In addition, you need to be familiar with the action, body parts, technique, number of times, facial expression, mental focus and breathing. It's worth noting that it takes time to be skillful in qigong practice. Consequently, you need to be determined, perseverant and persistent to remove disease and achieve health and longevity.

天 柱 导 引 功 · *Tian Zhu Dao Yin Gong*

Movements of *Tian Zhu Dao Yin Gong*

功法操作

本套功法包含了"天柱摆动法"与"三紧三松法"两大部分内容。

Tian Zhu Dao Yin Gong consists of Tian Zhu Swing exercise and three-intense and three-relaxed method.

天柱摆动法

Individual Movements of Tian Zhu Swing Exercise

第一势　顶天侧转拔天柱

Movement # 1　Lift the sky and turn the body to pull the spine

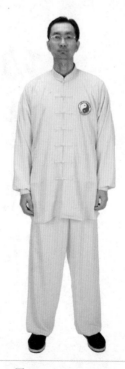

图 1-1-1　Fig 1-1-1

自然站直, 两足平行分开与肩同宽。

Stand upright, separate the feet to shoulder-width apart.

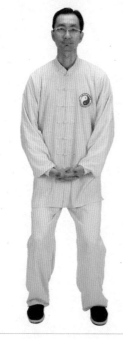

两手交叉，手心向上，落放在小腹，眼视正前方静心养息半分钟。

Cross the hands (palms forward) and place over the abdomen, look straight ahead and stay still for 30 seconds.

图 1-1-2　Fig 1-1-2

1. 吸气，两手沿着任脉上升至膻中反转，由内向外继续上升过头，两手仍交叉，手心顶天，两臂伸直贴近耳后方，百会顶天，要求虚领顶劲，两脚底沉地，形成两手心百会顶天，两脚底入地，其他肢体、躯干松弛，要求有拔天柱之感（图 1-1-3）。

1. Breathe in: Lift the hands along the Ren meridian[1] to Danzhong[2] (Ren 17), turn the hands outward and continue to lift above the top of the head. Lift the sky with the palms (of crossed hands), extend the arms to be close to the back of the ears and keep Baihui[3] (DU 20) upright.

[Tips]　Imagine a thread to connect the crown of the head (Baihui) to Dantian or pushing up energy and gently lead upward to the crown of the head (*Xu Ling Ding Jing*), touch the floor with the soles, lift the sky with the palms, relax the limbs and torso and feel the spine is pulled. (Fig 1-1-3)

---

1. One of the eight extraordinary meridians that travels along the front midline of the body.
2. Location: In the midline of the sternum, between the nipples level with the 4th intercostal space.
3. An acupuncture point located at the junction of a line connecting the apices of the ears (in the middle).

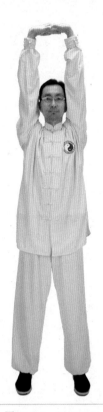

图 1-1-3　Fig 1-1-3

2. 呼气，身体由正前方向左旋转90°，两脚底不移动而沉地，尾骨沉地，两手顶天，百会顶天，其他肢体、躯干放松，要有拔天柱之感（图1-1-4）。

2. Breathe out: Turn 90° from straight ahead to the left, do not move the feet, sink the tailbone, lift the sky with the hands, keep Baihui (DU 20) upright, relax the limbs and torso and feel the spine is pulled. (Fig 1–1–4)

3. 吸气，身体由左方回转为正前方，两脚底不移动而沉地，两手心顶天，百会顶天，肢、躯干松弛，要有拔天柱之感。

3. Breathe in: Turn the body back to the neutral position, do not move the feet, sink the tailbone, lift the sky with the hands, keep Baihui (DU 20) upright, relax the limbs and torso and feel the spine is pulled.

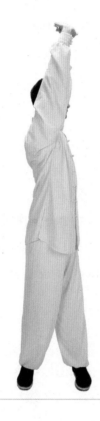

图 1-1-4　Fig 1-1-4

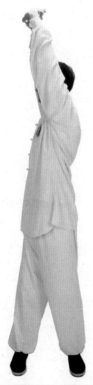

图 1-1-5　Fig 1-1-5

4. 呼气，身体由正前方，向右方向旋转90°，两脚底不移动而沉地，尾骨沉地，两手心顶天，百会顶天，其他肢、躯干放松，要有拔天柱之感（图1-1-5）。

4. Breathe out: Turn 90° from straight ahead to the right, do not move the feet, sink the tailbone, lift the sky with the hands, keep Baihui (DU 20) upright, relax the limbs and torso and feel the spine is pulled. (Fig 1-1-5)

5. 吸气，身体由右方，回转为正前方，两脚底不移动而沉地，尾骨沉地，两手心顶天，百会顶天，其他肢体、躯干放松，要有拔天柱之感。

5. Breathe in: Turn the body back to the neutral position, do not move the feet, sink the tailbone, lift the sky with the hands, keep Baihui (DU 20) upright, relax the limbs and torso and feel the spine is pulled.

6. 按照以上动作2、3、4、5左右旋转为1次，练习6~12次后收功。

6. 1 cycle contains 2, 3, 4 and 5, repeat 6-12 cycles.

7. 收功：身体在正前方姿势收功，把交叉顶天的两手自然松开，两手心由上向左右落下，两手心落放在大腿两侧，同时呼气，意念在小腹丹田部位，使小腹微微凸出，肢、躯干、头、颈、整体放松。这样肢体躯干练的气通过收功而回聚在丹田。

7. Concluding: Keep the body upright, release the crossed hands above the top of the head, and drop the hands to both sides of the thigh. Breathe out, focus the mental concentration on Dantian, slightly bulge the underbelly and relax the limbs, torso, head and neck. Through this, qi is returned to Dantian.

第二势　左右望月敲天柱

Movement # 2　Look at the moon from both sides and tap the spine

两足平行分开与肩宽，眼视正前方，站直，左右两手心撑腰部腰俞穴，意在两手心，松肩沉肘，静心养息半分钟。

Posture: Separate the feet to shoulder-width apart, look straight ahead, stand upright, place the palms on Yaoshu[1] (DU 2), focus the mental concentration on the palms, relax the shoulders, drop the elbows and stay still for 30 seconds.

1. 吸气，意在命门。

1. Breathe in: Focus the mental concentration on Mingmen[2].

2. 呼气，慢弯腰，抬头视前方，上身放松与地平行（图1–2–1）。

2. Breathe out: Slightly bend down, look upward and forward, relax the upper body and make the upper body parallel with the floor. (Fig 1–2–1)

3. 两掌变拳，用拳眼，轻轻敲打命门、腰椎、胸椎、尾间、夹脊等两侧，上下不停敲打1分钟（图1–2–2）。

3. Turn the palms into fists and gently tap both sides of Mingmen, lumbar vertebrae, thoracic vertebrae, coccyx, and Jiaji[3] points from top to bottom for 1 minute. (Fig 1–2–2)

---

1. An acupuncture point located in the sacral hiatus.
2. Mingmen literally means the gate of life, located between the kidneys, at the level of the second lumbar vertebrae.
3. A group of 34 points, 0.5 cun lateral to the lower border of the spinous processes from T1 to L5.

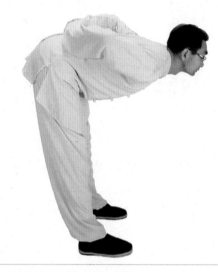

图 1-2-1　Fig 1-2-1

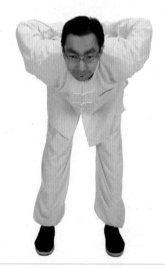

图 1-2-2　Fig 1-2-2

4. 呼气，上势不变，头由正位往左转后看到天上的星、月、日（图1-2-3、图1-2-4）。

4. Breathe out: Turn the head to left to look at the sky (star, moon and sun). (Fig 1–2–3, Fig 1–2–4)

---

5. 吸气，头回到原正位。

5. Breathe in: Return the head to the neutral position.

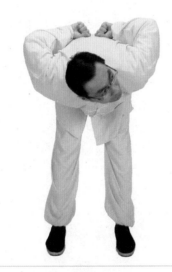

图 1–2–3　Fig 1–2–3

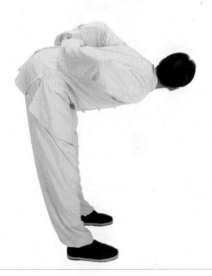

图 1–2–4　Fig 1–2–4

6. 呼气，头由正位往右转后看到天上的星、月、日（图1-2-5、图1-2-6）。

6. Breathe out: Turn the head to right to look at the sky (star, moon and sun). (Fig 1–2–5, Fig 1–2–6)

7. 吸气，头回到原正位。

7. Breathe in: Return the head to the neutral position.

8. 左右望月为1次，做3~6次。

8. One cycle consists of looking at the sky on both sides, and repeat 3–6 cycles.

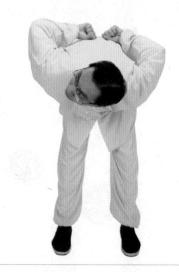

图 1-2-5　Fig 1-2-5

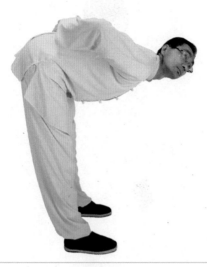

图 1-2-6 Fig 1-2-6

9. 呼气，沿着大腿、委中穴、小腿后敲打（图1-2-7、图1-2-8）。

9. Breathe out: Tap along the posterior aspect of the thigh, Weizhong[1] (BL 40) and lower leg. (Fig 1-2-7, Fig 1-2-8)

10. 吸气，沿着小腿外侧、足三里穴、大腿外侧至背部敲打（图1-2-9）。

10. Breathe in: Tap along the lateral side of the lower leg, Zusanli[2] (ST 36) and thigh until the back. (Fig 1-2-9)

---

1. An acupuncture point located at the center of the popliteal fossa.
2. An acupuncture point located on the anterior aspect of the lower leg, 3 cun below the depression lateral to the patella ligament, one finger-breadth (middle finger) from the anterior crest of the tibia.

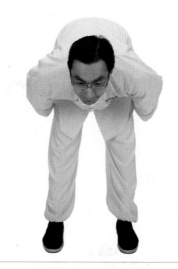

图 1-2-7　Fig 1-2-7

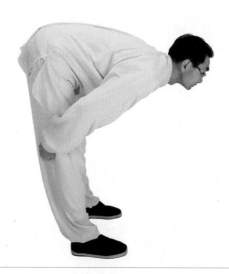

图 1-2-8　Fig 1-2-8

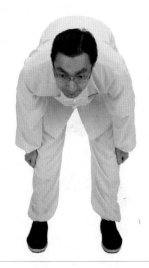

图 1-2-9　Fig 1-2-9

11. 重复动作9。

11. Repeat 9.

12. 重复动作10。

12. Repeat 10.

13. 两手垂落，继两手交叉，手心向天，松脱手腕、肘、肩、背、关节1分钟（图1-2-10、图1-2-11）。

13. Drop the hands, cross the hands and lift the sky with the palms, relax the wrist, elbows, shoulders and joint for 1 minute. (Fig 1-2-10, Fig 1-2-11)

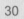
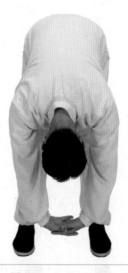

图 1-2-10　Fig 1-2-10

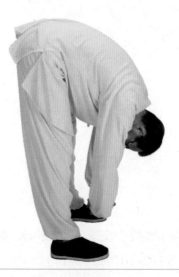

图 1-2-11　Fig 1-2-11

14. 继上两手交叉，手心由内向下转向正前方，两上肢伸直，肩关节放松，身体下蹲（图1-2-12、图1-2-13）。

14. Turn the palms (from inward to downward) straight forward, extend the upper limbs, relax the shoulders and squat down. (Fig 1-2-12, Fig 1-2-13)

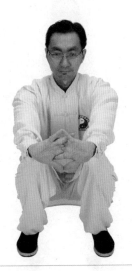

图 1-2-12　Fig 1-2-12

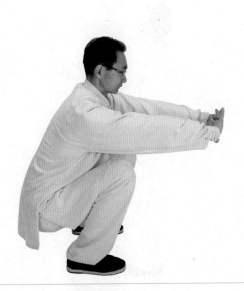

图 1-2-13　Fig 1-2-13

15. 吸气，身体缓缓站起再下沉形成站桩势，上肢不变，形成虎背式站桩（图1-2-14、图1-2-15）。

15. Breathe in: Slowly stand up and squat down to a *Zhan Zhuang* posture (tiger back) (Fig 1–2–14, Fig 1–2–15)

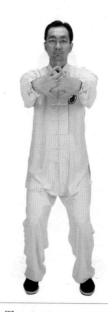
图 1-2-14　Fig 1–2–14

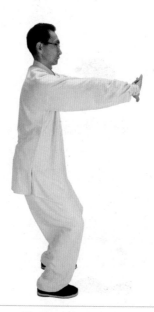

图 1-2-15　Fig 1–2–15

16. 虎背式站桩：两足平行分开与肩宽，两膝不过脚尖，落腰收胯，腰椎伸直，两手交叉(两大指、两小指相触)，手心向前，肘关节伸直，沉肩、松肩、虚领顶劲，含胸拔背，两眼视两小指间前方，半分钟后闭眼，用意视两小指间前，交替进行数分钟。

16. Tiger back standing (*Zhan Zhuang*): Separate the feet to shoulder-width apart, do not let the knees go past the toes, relax the waist and hips and straighten the lumbar vertebrae. Cross the hands (let the thumbs and little fingers touch each other) with palms forward, extend the elbow joints and drop and relax the shoulders. Imagine a thread to connect the crown of the head (Baihui) to Dantian (*Xu Ling Ding Jing*), tuck in the chest and pull up the back. Focus the eyes on the space between little fingers, close the eyes in 30 seconds and focus the mental concentration on the space between little fingers. Repeat alternately for a couple of minutes.

17. 收功：吸气两手臂放松，上举托天，两脚自然伸直。

17. Concluding: Breathe in, release the arms and lift to support the sky and extend the legs.

18. 呼气，意在丹田，小腹逐渐微凸，两手心向左右外、向下至落放在两大腿外侧。

18. Breathe out, focus the mental concentration on Dantian, Slowly and slightly bulge the belly, turn the palms outward, downward and drop the hands to bilateral sides of the thigh.

第三势　左右侧弯弓天柱

Movement # 3　Bend to left and right to pull the spine

两足平行分开比肩宽，两脚自然站直，两手落放在两大腿外侧，做到沉肩垂指，眼视正前方，意在小腹丹田，静心养息半分钟。

Posture: Separate the feet to shoulder-width apart, stand upright, and place the hands to bilateral sides of the thigh. Drop the shoulders and fingers, look straight ahead, focus the mental concentration on Dantian and stay still for 30 seconds.

1. 吸气，左手从左侧上举，手心向左外侧，左上臂贴耳，肘关节伸直，指尖顶天（图1-3-1）。

1. Breath in: Lift the left hand from the left side, turn the left palm outward and let the left upper arm close to the ear. Extend the elbow and make the fingers pointing upward. (Fig 1-3-1)

2. 呼气，右手中指沿着右腿中间摸着裤缝向下，弯腰摸至右膝关节左右，左上臂贴在左耳不变（图1-3-2）。

2. Breathe out: Use the middle finger of the right hand to slide down along the trouser seam, bend to the right knee, and do not move the left upper arm. (Fig 1-3-2)

3. 吸气，两手往右外侧方向伸，腰逐步变直，两手上举，两手心向前，手指顶天（图1-3-3）。

3. Breathe in: Extend both hands to the right side, slowly straighten up the waist and lift the hands, with palms forward and fingers pointing upward. (Fig 1-3-3)

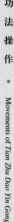

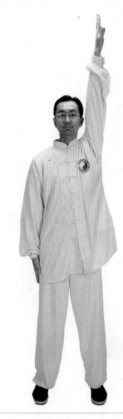

图 1-3-1　Fig 1-3-1

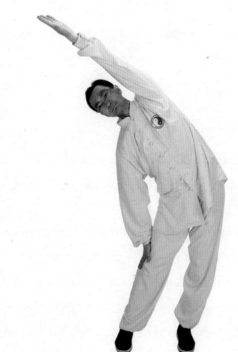

图 1-3-2　Fig 1-3-2

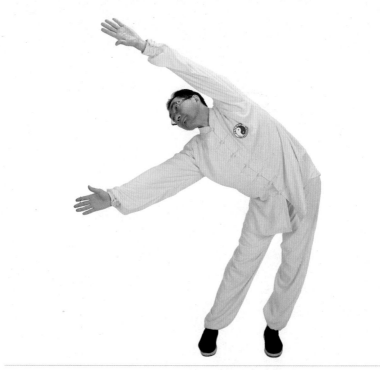

图 1-3-3　Fig 1-3-3

4. 呼气, 两手自然垂落, 往左外侧转下, 手指垂地, 两手心向大腿(图1-3-4)。

4. Breathe out: Drop the hands naturally and turn upper left, with the fingers pointing downward and the palms facing the thigh. (Fig 1-3-4)

5. 吸气, 两手自然伸直、往右外侧、转上, 右上臂贴右耳、肘关节伸直、指尖顶天、手心向右、左手继向左外侧、向下、落放在左大腿外侧、中指贴裤缝(图1-3-5)。

5. Breathe in: Extend the hands and turn right upward and let the right upper arm close to the ear. Extend the elbow and make the fingers point upward and the palms face right. Turn the left hand to lower left, drop the left hand to the lateral side of the left thigh and place the middle finger on the trouser seam. (Fig 1-3-5)

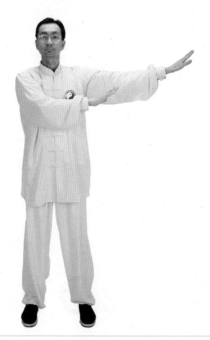

图 1-3-4　Fig 1-3-4

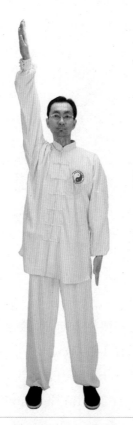

图 1-3-5　Fig 1-3-5

6. 呼气, 左侧弯、左手中指沿着裤缝下去至左膝关节左右, 右手上臂贴右耳不变(图 1-3-6)。

6. Breathe out: Use the middle finger of the left hand to slide down along the trouser seam, bend to the left knee, and do not move the right upper arm. (Fig 1-3-6)

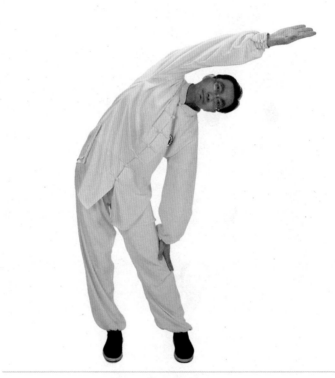

图 1-3-6 Fig 1-3-6

7. 吸气, 两手往左侧外方向伸, 腰逐步复直, 两手上举, 两手心向前, 手指顶天(图 1-3-7)。

7. Breathe in: Extend both hands to the left side, slowly straighten up the waist and lift the hands, with palms forward and fingers pointing upward. (Fig 1-3-7)

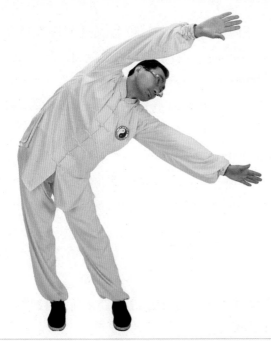

图 1-3-7   Fig 1-3-7

8. 呼气，两手自然伸直，往右外侧转下、垂地，两手心向大腿（图1-3-8）。

8. Breathe out: Extend and turn the hands lower right to touch the floor, with the palms facing the thighs. (Fig 1-3-8)

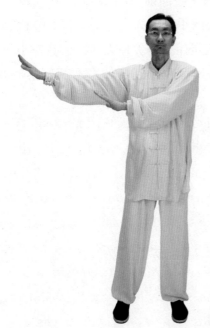

图 1-3-8   Fig 1-3-8

9. 吸气，两手自然伸直、往左外侧、转上、左上臂贴左耳、肘关节伸直、指尖顶天、手心向左，右手继向右外侧、向下、落放在右大腿外侧、中指贴裤缝。

9. Breathe in: Extend and turn the hands to upper left. Let the left upper arm close to the left ear and extend the elbow with the fingers pointing upward and the palms facing left. Drop the right hand to lower right until the lateral side of the right thigh and place the middle finger on the trouser seam.

10. 自动作2至动作9左右侧弯为1次，要求练6~12次，刚开始练习时可逐步增加次数。

10. One cycle includes 2–9. Repeat 6–12 cycles and gradually increase the frequency.

11. 收功：接动作7吸气，右手、左手往左外侧方向伸、腰逐步复直、两手上举、两手心向前，手指顶天。呼气，两手自然伸直、往右侧转下垂地、两手心向大腿。吸气，两手继续向左外侧、向上，两手上举、手心向前、手尖顶天，呼气，意在小腹丹田、腹略前凸、形成气沉丹田。两手在身体左右两侧落放在大腿外侧。

11. Concluding: Further to 7 breathe in, extend the hands to the left, slowly straighten up the waist and lift the hands, with palms forward and fingers pointing upward. Breathe out, extend the hands and turn right downward to touch the floor, with the palms facing the thigh. Breathe in, continue to turn the hands left upward and lift the hands, with the palms facing the thigh and fingers pointing upward. Breathe out, focus the mental concentration on Dantian, slightly bulge the belly and let qi sink to Dantian. Drop the hands to both sides of the thighs.

第四势　前弯后仰转天柱

Movement # 4　Bend forward and lean backward to rotate the spine

两足平行分开与肩同宽，自然站立、沉肩垂指、眼视正前方，深呼吸3次。

Posture: Separate the feet to shoulder-width apart and stand naturally. Relax the shoulders, drop the fingers, look straight ahead and take three times of deep breath.

1. 吸气，两手自然伸直由前至上举、指尖顶天、手心向前（图1–4–1）。

1. Breathe in: Extend the hands forward and lift with the fingers pointing upward and the palms forward. (Fig 1–4–1)

2. 呼气，前弯腰，两手由前向下至手指触地，脚跟似离地非离地（图1–4–2）。

2. Breathe out: Bend forward and drop the hands to touch the floor with fingers, with a feeling of heels off the floor. (Fig 1–4–2)

3. 吸气，两手前伸上举随躯体直起至后仰，手心向天，两手前伸时脚跟似离地非离地（图1–4–3）。

3. Breathe in: Extend the hands forward with a feeling of heels off the floor. Lift the hands along with straightening up of the body and then lean backward with the palms upward. (Fig 1–4–3)

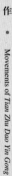
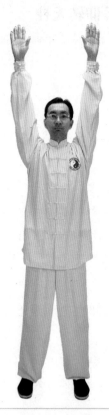

图 1-4-1　Fig 1-4-1

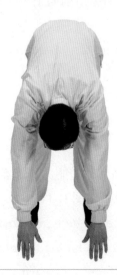

图 1-4-2　Fig 1-4-2

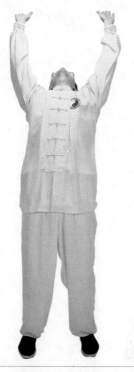

图 1-4-3 Fig 1-4-3

4. 呼气，身、头、手慢慢左转90°，至腰伸直，继左右各转30°各2次至复正位，要求上肢、肩放松（图1-4-4、图1-4-5、图1-4-6）。

4. Breathe out: Slowly turn the body, head and hand 90° to the left until the waist is straightened up. Then turn 30° to left and right (twice on each side) and return to a neutral position. It's essential to relax the upper limbs and shoulders. (Fig 1–4–4, Fig 1–4–5, Fig 1–4–6)

5. 深吸气，姿势不变。

5. Deep inhalation: Do not change the posture.

6. 呼气，前弯腰、两手由前向下至手指触地、脚跟似要离地。

6. Breathe out: Bend forward, drop the hands to touch the floor with the fingers, with a feeling of heels off the floor.

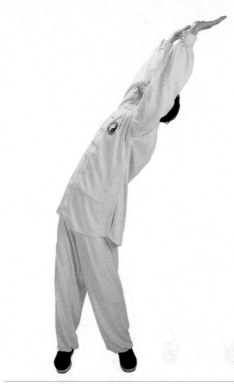

图 1-4-4　Fig 1-4-4

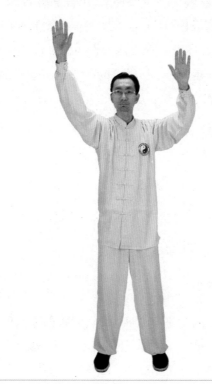

图 1-4-5　Fig 1-4-5

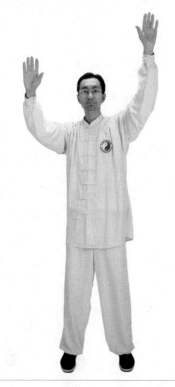

图 1-4-6　Fig 1-4-6

7. 吸气，身体慢慢伸直至后弯、面仰天、两手前伸继上举至后仰、手心向天，手在前伸时，脚跟似要离地。

7. Breathe in: Slowly straighten the body and lean backward with face up. Extend the hands forward with a feeling of heels off the floor. Then lift and lean backward, with the palms upward.

8. 呼气，身、头、手慢慢右转90°至腰伸直，继左右各转30°，各2次至复正位。要求上肢、肩放松（图1-4-7）。

8. Breathe out: Slowly turn the body, head and hand 90° to the right until the waist is straightened up. Then turn 30° to left and right (twice on each side) and return to a neutral position. It's essential to relax the upper limbs and shoulders. (Fig 1-4-7)

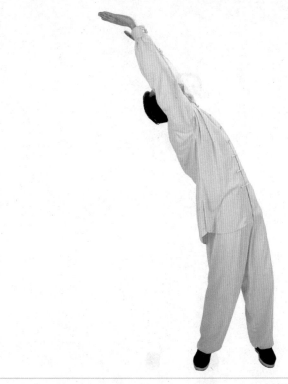

图 1-4-7   Fig 1-4-7

9. 动作2至动作8为1次,练6~12次。

9. One cycle includes 4.2–4.8, repeat 6–12 cycles.

10. 收功:接动作8深吸气、意在腹部丹田、姿势不变。呼气,意在腹部丹田、并微微凸起,两手由身体两侧下落,落放在大腿外侧。

10. Concluding: Further to 8, take a deep breath, focus the mental concentration on Dantian and keep the posture. Breathe out, focus the mental concentration on Dantian, slightly bulge the belly. Drop the hands to both sides of the thighs.

［注意］动作由小到大,调身逐步正确,呼吸自然,身心舒畅。

［Tips］ Increase the movement amplitude gradually and breathe naturally.

三紧三松法

Individual Movements of Three-Intense and Three-Relaxed Method

三紧法
Three-intense exercise

第一势　前倾站桩往后瞧
Movement # 1　Stand with upper body forward to look back

1. 两足平行分开与肩同宽、两手心撑在左右腰部肾俞穴、两肘关节往后、挺胸、百会顶天、下额后收、眼视前方、意在命门、静心养息半分钟（图2–1–1）。

1. Separate the feet to shoulder-width apart and place the palms on bilateral Shenshu[1] (BL 23). Pull the elbows backward, chest out, keep Baihui (DU 20) upright and tuck in the chin. Look straight ahead, focus the mental concentration on Mingmen and stay still for 30 seconds. (Fig 2–1–1)

2. 呼气，上身慢慢前倾，两眼视地离脚尖4米，身体的重心移到涌泉穴位，足跟似要离地。

---

1. An acupuncture point located below the spinous process of the 2nd lumbar vertebra, 1.5 cun lateral to the posterior midline.

2. Breathe out: Slowly bend the upper body forward, focus the eyes on the floor (4 meters away from the tiptoe) and shift the body weight to Yongquan[1] (KI 1), with a feeling of heels off the floor.

3. 吸气，收腰，提肛，提外肾，提内脏。

3. Breathe in: Tighten the waist and lift up the anus, testicles and internal organs.

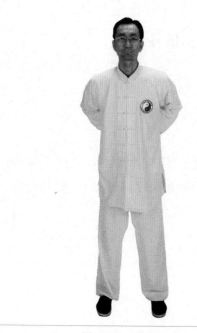

图 2-1-1　Fig 2-1-1

1. An acupuncture point located on the sole, in the depression appearing on the anterior part of the sole when the foot is in the plantar flexion, approximately at the junction of the anterior third and posterior two thirds of the line connecting the base of the 2nd and 3rd toes and the heel.

4. 呼气, 身体、四肢、姿势不变, 头往左后方向, 眼视地保持离脚尖4米处往左后方向移, 做到松肛、松外肾、松内脏（图2-1-2）。

4. Breathe out: Do not move the body and four limbs. Turn the head to left rear, focus the eyes on the floor and move to left rear, and relax the anus, testicles and internal organs. (Fig 2-1-2)

5. 吸气, 收腰, 提肛, 提外肾, 提内脏, 头复正前, 眼视离脚尖4米地面, 复回正前。

5. Breathe in: Tighten the waist and lift up the anus, testicles and internal organs. Return the head to a neutral position and focus the eyes on the floor (4 meters away from the tiptoe) and return to look straight ahead.

6. 呼气, 身体、四肢、姿势不变, 头往右后方向, 眼视地保持离

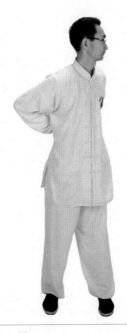

图 2-1-2　Fig 2-1-2

脚尖4米处，往右后方向移，做到松肛，松外肾，松内脏（图2-1-3）。

6. Breathe out: Do not move the body and four limbs. Turn the head to right rear, focus the eyes on the floor (4 meters away from the tiptoe) and move to right rear, and relax the anus, testicles and internal organs. (Fig 2–1–3)

7. 吸气，收腰，提肛，提外肾，提内脏，头复正前，眼视离脚尖4米地面，复回正前（图2-1-4）。

7. Breathe in: Tighten the waist and lift up the anus, testicles and internal organs. Return the head to a neutral position and focus the eyes on the floor (4 meters away from the tiptoe) and return to look straight ahead. (Fig 2–1–4)

8. 动作4至动作7左右后转为1次，做6~12次。

8. One cycle includes 4–7, repeat 6–12 cycles.

9. 收功：接动作7，呼气，上身前倾姿势慢慢恢复自然站立，两手下至环跳、下落在大腿外侧，整肢体放松，意在腹部，气沉丹田。

9. Concluding: Further to 7, breathe out, slowly stand upright from forward bending of the upper body, and drop the hands to Huantiao[1] (GB 30) and bilateral sides of the thighs. Relax the body, focus the mental concentration on the abdomen and let qi sink to Dantian.

---

1. An acupuncture point located on the lateral side of the thigh, at the junction of the middle third and lateral third of the line connecting the prominence of the great trochanter and the sacral hiatus when the patient is in a lateral recumbent position with the thigh flexed.

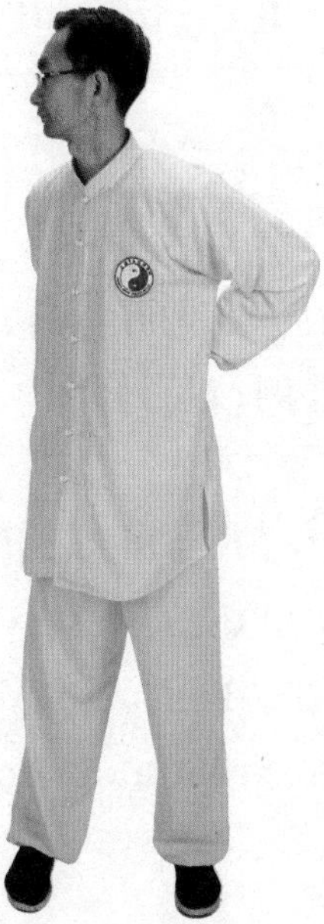

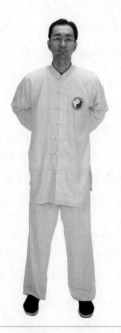

图 2-1-3　Fig 2-1-3

图 2-1-4　Fig 2-1-4

第二势 吐纳导引理三焦

Movement # 2　Exhale and inhale to regulate *Sanjiao*

　　两脚平行分开与肩同宽，两膝弯曲、膝关节不超过足尖，两手自然落放在两大腿外侧，口目轻闭，意在涌泉，静心养息半分钟。

Posture: Separate the feet to shoulder-width apart, bend at the knees and do not let the knees go past the toes. Drop the hands to both sides of the thighs, slightly close the mouth and eyes, focus the mental concentration on Yongquan (KI 1), and stay still for 30 seconds.

　　1. 吸气，两手上提在胯两侧形成握拳、拳心向上，两脚自然伸直，意从涌泉穴→腹部丹田（图2-2-1）。

1. Breathe in: Lift the hands to the hips and turn into fists (pointing upward), extend the feet and focus the mental concentration from Yongquan (KI 1) to abdominal Dantian. (Fig 2-2-1)

　　2. 呼气，松拳，中指相触，手心向上放在小腹前，两膝慢慢弯曲、膝不超过足尖，躯体垂地下沉，意从丹田→涌泉穴（图2-2-2）。

2. Breathe out: Release the fists, let the middle fingers of both hands touch each other, and place the hands with palms upward in front of the abdomen. Slightly bend the knees (do not let the knees go past the toes), lower down the body and focus the mental concentration from Dantian to Yongquan (KI 1). (Fig 2-2-2)

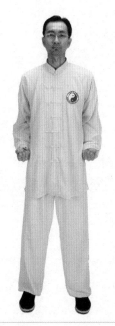

图 2-2-1　Fig 2-2-1

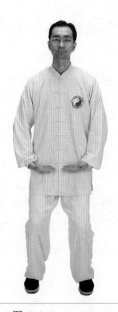

图 2-2-2　Fig 2-2-2

3. 吸气，两手慢慢上提近膻中，两脚自然伸直，意从涌泉穴→丹田→膻中（图2-2-3）。

3. Breathe in: Slowly lift the hands to Danzhong[1] (Ren 17), extend the feet and focus the mental concentration from Yongquan (KI 1) → Dantian → Danzhong (Ren 17). (Fig 2-2-3)

4. 呼气，两手心向身→向地→向外→向上→伸臂→托天，虎口相对，掌有托天之力，意从膻中→内劳宫穴位开眼看天，脚跟离地（图2-2-4）。

4. Breathe out: Turn the palms inward → outward → upward → to lift the sky with the palms, making the *Hukou* (space between the thumb and index finger) area facing each other. Focus the mental concentration from Danzhong (Ren 17) to Laogong[2] (PC 8). Then open the eyes to look up to the sky, with heels off the floor. (Fig 2-2-4)

5. 吸气，两手转掌慢慢下降至膻中，脚跟着地，意在两内宫穴→膻中穴（图2-2-5）。

5. Breathe in: Slowly drop the hands to Danzhong (Ren 17), touch the floor with the heels and focus the mental concentration from bilateral Laogong (PC 8) to Danzhong (Ren 7). (Fig 2-2-5)

6. 呼气，闭眼两手慢慢下降至小腹，手心向下，两膝弯曲、不超过足尖，身体垂地下沉，意从膻中→丹田→涌泉。

6. Breathe out: Close the eyes and slowly drop the hands

---

1. An acupuncture point located at the level with the 4th intercostal space, midway between the nipples.
2. An acupuncture point located at the centre of the palm, between the 2nd and 3rd metacarpal bones, but close to the latter, and in the part touching the tip of the middle finger when a fist is made.

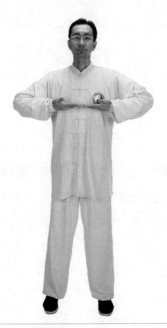

图 2-2-3　Fig 2-2-3

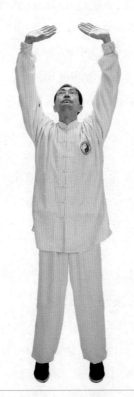

图 2-2-4　Fig 2-2-4

to the lower abdomen, with the palms downward. Slightly bend at the knees (do not let the knees go past the toes), lower the body and focus the mental concentration from Danzhong (Ren 17) → Dantian → Yongquan (KI 1).

7. 吸气，两手心→向身→向上→握拳移放在胯部，拳心向上，两膝自然伸直，意从涌泉→丹田（图2-2-6）。

7. Breathe in: Turn the palms inward → upward → into fists (pointing upward) and place on the hips. Extend the knees and focus the mental concentration from Yongquan (KI 1) to Dantian. (Fig 2-2-6)

8. 呼气，松拳，手心→向腿→向地，两上肢自然伸直，躯体垂地下沉，膝关节弯曲、不超过足尖，意从丹田→涌泉。

8. Breathe out: Release the fists and turn the palms facing the leg and then downward. Extend the upper limbs, lower the body, bend at the knees (do not let the knees go past the toes) and focus the mental concentration from Dantian to Yongquan (KI 1).

9. 动作1至动作8为1次，练6～12次。

9. One cycle includes 1 to 8, repeat 6–12 cycles.

10. 收功：接动作8吸气，两下肢自然站直、两手心微碰大腿外侧。意在丹田，慢慢睁开两眼。

10. Concluding: Further to 2.8, breathe in, straighten up the lower limbs, slightly touch the bilateral sides of the thighs with the palms, focus the mental concentration on Dantian and slowly open the eyes.

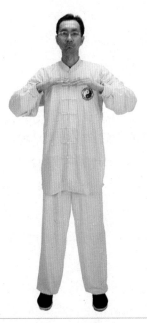

图 2-2-5　Fig 2-2-5

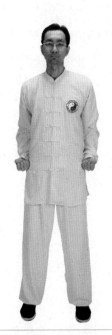

图 2-2-6　Fig 2-2-6

第三势　单脚下蹲壮筋气

Movement # 3　Squat on one foot to strengthen the tendons

1. 左脚虚在前,右脚实在后的站桩。两脚平行分开小于肩宽,左脚向正前方移半个脚印,形成左脚虚在前、右脚实在后的站桩,腰椎自然伸直,含胸拔背、虚领顶劲,松肩垂肘,腋中空松,手心向地,意念在两手心似按水球各一同时似想丹田,口目轻闭,脸带笑容,呼吸自然,练半分钟至3分钟(图2-3-1)。

收功:吸气意在丹田,两脚自然伸直,两手靠拢在大腿外侧,睁眼。

1. Stand with unweighted left foot forward and weighted right foot backward: Separate the feet narrower than should-width and move the left foot half a step straight ahead to stand with unweighted left foot forward and weighted right foot backward. Straighten up the lumbar spine, tuck in the chest, pull up the back, and imagine a thread to connect the crown of the head (Baihui) to Dantian. Relax the shoulders and drop the elbows (a hollow, loosened armpit). With the palms downward, imagine pressing an inflated balloon in water with the palms, and focus mental concentration on Dantian. Slightly close the mouth and eyes, smile, breathe naturally and stay for 30 seconds to 3 minutes. (Fig 2-3-1)

Concluding: Breathe in, focus the mental concentration on Dantian, extend the feet, drop the hands to bilateral sides of the thighs and open the eyes.

2. 右脚虚在前、左脚实在后的站桩。调身、调息、调心、收功同上(图2-3-2)。

2. Stand with unweighted right foot forward and weighted

left foot backward. Then perform same regulation of the body, breathing and mind and conclude as 1. (Fig 2–3–2)

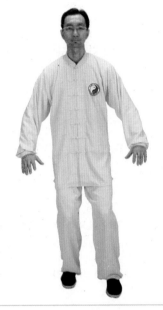

图 2-3-1　Fig 2-3-1

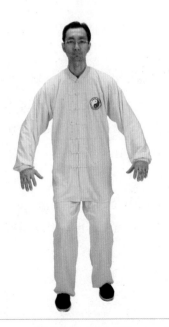

图 2-3-2　Fig 2-3-2

三松法
Three-relaxed exercise

第一势　拍打肩并理首躯
Movement # 1　Tap the shoulders to regulate the head and torso

两足平行分开小于肩宽、两膝微弯,眼视前方,直腰拔背,下颌后收、百会顶天,两手自然落放在大腿外侧。

Posture: Separate the feet narrower than shoulder-width apart, bend at the knees, and look straight ahead. Straighten the waist, pull up the back, tuck in the chin, keep Baihui (DU 20) upright and drop the hands to bilateral sides of the thighs.

1. 腰胯向左转动,两脚底着地,脸部向前不变,甩动两上肢,右手大鱼际外侧拍打左肩井,左手背拍打背部,要求两手同时各拍打着肩井和背部位时短粗呼气,意在拍打的部位放松(图3-1-1、图3-1-2)。

1. Turn the waist and hip to the left, touch the floor with the soles and keep the face forward. Swing the upper limbs, use the lateral side of the thenar eminence of the right hand to tap Jianjin[1] (GB 21) and use the dorsum of the left hand to tap the back. (Fig 3-1-1, Fig 3-1-2)

［Tips］ Exhale short and fast while tapping Jianjin (GB 21) and the back simultaneously with both hands (to relax the local area).

---

1. An acupuncture point located on the shoulder directly above the nipple at the midpoint of a line connecting the spinous process of C7 and the acromion.

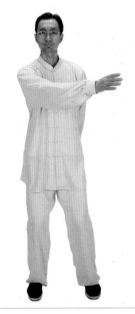

图 3-1-1　Fig 3-1-1

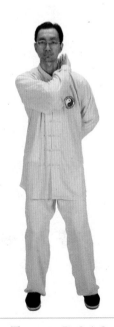

图 3-1-2　Fig 3-1-2

2. 腰胯向右动，两脚底着地不变，整脸向前不变，甩动两上肢、左手大鱼际外侧拍打右肩井、右手背拍打背部，要求两手同时各拍打着肩井和背部位时短粗呼气，意在拍打的部位放松（图3-1-3、图3-1-4），练50~100次。

2. Move the waist and hip to the right and do not move the soles and face. Swing the upper limbs, use the lateral side of the thenar eminence of the left hand to tap Jianjin[1] (GB 21) and use the dorsum of the right hand to tap the back. (Fig 3-1-3, Fig 3-1-4)

［Tips］ Exhale short and fast while tapping Jianjin (GB 21) and the back simultaneously with both hands (to relax the local area)

Repeat 50–100 times.

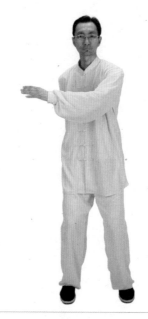

图 3-1-3　Fig 3-1-3

1. An acupuncture point located on the shoulder directly above the nipple at the midpoint of a line connecting the spinous process of C7 and the acromion.

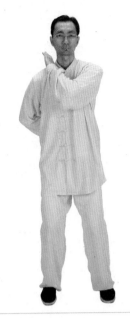

图 3-1-4　　Fig 3-1-4

第二势　拍打曲池祛瘀滞
Movement # 2　Tap Quchi[1] (LI 11) to resolve stagnation

　　两脚平行分开与肩同宽，两膝自然弯曲，眼看前方，两手落放在大腿外侧，手指向下。

　　Posture: Separate the feet to shoulder-width apart, naturally bend at the knees and look straight ahead. Drop the hands to bilateral sides of the thighs, with fingers pointing downward.

　　1. 左手向右→向上→向左→向下转近一圈，右手随着向右→向上→向左→向下转近一圈，右手小鱼际外侧与左肢曲池穴相击，左手心即拍在右肘关节外侧，用鼻短粗呼气，意默念松字（图3-2-1、

---

1. An acupuncture point located at the lateral end of the transverse cubital crease midway between cubital crease (radial side of the tendon of m. biceps brachii) and the lateral epicondyle of the humerus.

图3-2-2、图3-2-3）。

1. Turn the left hand → right → upward → left → downward and turn the right hand → right → upward → left downward. Use the lateral side of the thenar eminence of the right hand to strike Quchi[1] (LI 11) on the left arm, use the left palm to tap the lateral side of the right elbow, exhale short and fast and aspirate the sound of '*Song*' silently. (Fig 3-2-1, Fig 3-2-2, Fig 3-2-3)

身体向右→向左自然随左手转动，左手向上时，两下肢自然伸直，左手向下时，两下肢自然弯曲。

Turn the body → right → left with the left hand. Extend the lower limbs while lifting the left hand and flex the lower limbs while dropping the left hand.

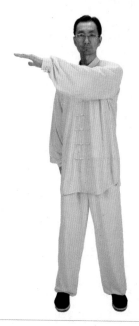

图 3-2-1　Fig 3-2-1

---

1. An acupuncture point located at (with the elbow flexed) the lateral end of the cubital crease (radial side of the tendon of m. biceps brachii) and external humeral epicondyle.

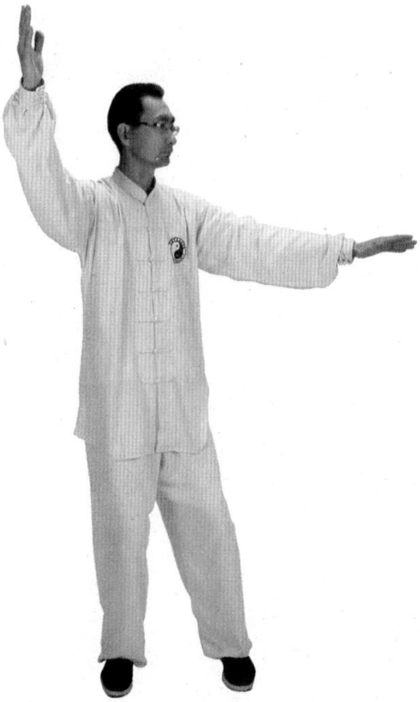

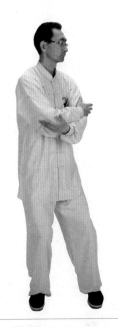

图 3-2-2　Fig 3-2-2

图 3-2-3　Fig 3-2-3

2. 右手向左→向上→向右→向下转近一圈，左手随着向左→向上→向右→向下转近一圈，左手小鱼际外侧与右肢曲池穴相击，右手心即拍在左肘关节外侧，鼻短粗呼气，意默念松字（图3-2-4、图3-2-5）。

2. Turn the right hand → left → upward → right → downward and turn the left hand → left → upward → right → downward. Use the lateral side of the hypothenar eminence of the left hand to strike Quchi (LI 11) on the right arm, use the right palm to tap the lateral side of the left elbow, exhale short and fast and aspirate the sound of '*Song*' silently. (Fig 3-2-4, Fig 3-2-5)

身体向左→向右自然随右手转动，右手向上时两下肢自然伸直，右手向下时两下肢自然弯曲，一左一右为1次，练20~50次。

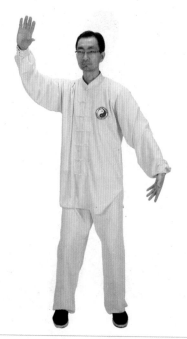

图 3-2-4　Fig 3-2-4

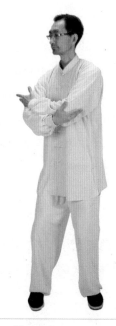

图 3-2-5   Fig 3-2-5

Turn the boby → left → right with the right hand. Extend the lower limbs while lifting the right hand and flex the lower limbs while dropping the right hand.

Repeat 30–50 times on each side.

3. 收功：接动作2吸气，两手上举，两侧下落，两脚自然伸直，意在丹田；呼气，两手从身两侧落放在大腿旁，意整体放松，气沉丹田。

3. Concluding: Further to 2.2, breathe in, lift the hands, extend the feet and focus the mental concentration on Dantian. Breathe out, drop the hands to bilateral sides of the thighs, relax the body and let qi sink to Dantian.

第三势　拍打胯部理躯肢

Movement # 3　Tap the hips to regulate torso and limbs

两脚平行分开比肩宽，两膝微弯，腰背自然伸直，眼视前方，两手落放在大腿外侧，静心平气半分钟。

Posture: Separate the fee to shoulder-width apart, slightly bend at the knees and straighten up the waist and back. Look straight ahead, drop the hands to bilateral sides of the thighs and stay still for 30 seconds.

1. 两手小鱼际拍打腹股沟4次→胯外侧4次→胯后外侧4次→胯外侧4次→腹股沟4次为1次，练5～10次（图3-3-1、图3-3-2、图3-3-3）。

1. Use the hypothenar eminences of both hands to tap groin 4 times → bilateral sides of the hips 4 times → posterior-lateral sides of the hips 4 times → bilateral sides of the thighs 4

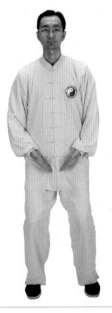

图 3-3-1　Fig 3-3-1

times → groin 4 times. Repeat this procedure 5–10 times. (Fig 3–3–1, Fig 3–3–2, Fig 3–3–3)

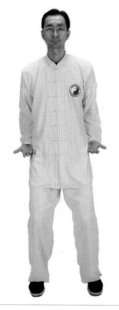

图 3–3–2　Fig 3–3–2

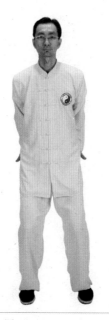

图 3–3–3　Fig 3–3–3

2. 两手心面拍大腿前4次→外侧4次→环跳4次→外侧4次→大腿前4次为1次，练5～10次（图3-3-4、图3-3-5、图3-3-6）。

2. Use the palms to tap anterior aspect of the thigh 4 times → lateral side of the thigh 4 times → Huantiao (GB 30) 4 times → lateral side of the thigh 4 times anterior aspect of the thigh 4 times. Repeat this procedure 5–10 times. (Fig 3–3–4, Fig 3–3–5, Fig 3–3–6)

3. 大腿外侧→小腿外侧方向拍，速度一寸一寸往下移（拍打足三里部位时为10～20秒）（图3-3-7）。

3. Tap from bilateral sides of the thighs to bilateral sides of the lower leg, move down one cun by one cun → tap Zusanli (ST 36) 10–20 seconds. (Fig 3–3–7)

4. 小腿外侧→大腿外侧方向拍，速度一寸一寸往上移（拍打足三里部位时为10～20秒）。

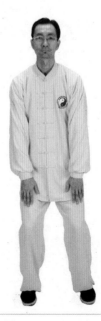

图 3-3-4　Fig 3-3-4

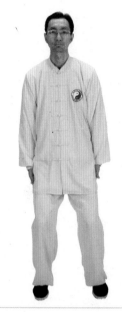

图 3-3-5　Fig 3-3-5

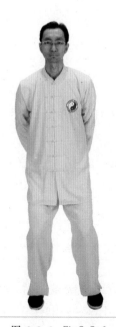

图 3-3-6　Fig 3-3-6

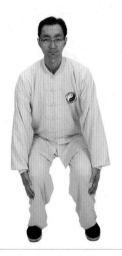

图 3-3-7　Fig 3-3-7

4. Tap from bilateral sides of the lower leg to bilateral sides of the thighs move up one cun by one cun → tap Zusanli (ST 36) 10–20 seconds.

5. 重复动作1、2。

5. Repeat 3.1 and 3.2

6. 收功：吸气，两脚自然伸直，两手落放在大腿外侧、意在丹田。

6. Concluding: Breathe in, extend the feet, drop the hands to bilateral sides of the thighs and focus the mental concentration on Dantian.

［注意］三紧三松法，要松紧结合，意不能在头部。拍打到局部时，意念要放松，并用鼻短粗呼气，身体左右转动自然，根据练功者的体质增加锻炼次数。

［Tips］ It's important to combine intense exercises with

relaxation method. Do not keep the mental focus on the head. Relax mental focus when tapping local body parts. Exhale short and fast with the nose, naturally turn the body and increase exercise frequencies according to individual constitution.

天 柱 导 引 功　·　*Tian Zhu Dao Yin Gong*

Application

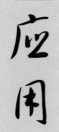

本功法是传统导引功法,通过肢体的伸缩导引,配合呼吸、意识的运用,有如下的功效与作用。

As a traditional *Dao Yin* exercise, *Tian Zhu Dao Yin Gong* involves body movements, breathing and mental concentration. Its functions are as follows:

疏 通 经 络

Unblocks meridians

经络是气血运行的通路。经络不通则痛,脏腑组织器官得不到气血的滋养和温煦,导致各种病症。通过本功法的习练可有效促进经络疏通,如天柱摆动法可疏通两侧胆经和督脉,同时也疏通背后膀胱经,使全身阳气舒畅;三紧三松法能疏通肾经、脾经、胃经与任督两脉等。经络通则不痛,脏腑组织就能得到濡养和舒解。

Meridians are pathways of qi and blood circulation. Blockage of meridians causes pain and malnourishment of zang-fu organs and tissues. This exercise can unblock meridians. Specifically, *Tian Zhu* swing exercise can regulate gallbladder, Du and bladder meridians and activate yang qi of the entire body, and three-intense and three-relaxed method can regulate kidney, spleen, stomach, Ren, and Du meridians. Unblocking of meridians relieves pain and other zang-fu problems.

调　和　气　血

Harmonizes qi and blood

气血是滋养人体的营养物质。如果气血不足就可导致贫血或营养不良，免疫功能下降，就产生许多虚证病候；如果气滞血瘀就可导致气血运行障碍，会产生许多实证病候。通过习练本功法，特别是其中的站桩功，能增强腿脚的实力，长劲、长气、长力，不仅可以补益气血，而且又可理气活血，所以能够防治各种虚证和实证等许多病症。

Qi and blood nurture the body. Insufficient qi and blood may cause anemia, malnutrition, weakened immune system and deficiency syndrome. Qi stagnation and blood stasis may cause excess syndrome. This exercise, especially the *Zhan Zhuang*, can strengthen the legs and feet, supplement and regulate qi, tonify and circulation blood. As a result, it can be used for both deficiency syndrome and excess syndrome.

伸　筋　拔　骨

Stretches the tendons/bones

通过本功法习练，特别是天柱摆动法的习练，可以让脊柱进行旋转、屈曲、侧弯以及伸展等不同的运动，充分锻炼人体平时不太活动的肌肉、韧带和小关节等，能够起到伸筋拔骨、通利关节的作用，另外还能锻炼腿后及背上的大筋，并进而激发脏腑的腧穴，调节脏腑气血与功能，以达到养生健体的功效。

This exercise, especially Tian Zhu swing exercise involves the rotation, flexion, lateral bending and stretching of the spine. It can therefore work on muscles, ligaments and facet joints that we do not often exercise, and thus stretch tendons and bones and benefit joints. In addition, it can work on large tendons on the back and posterior aspect of the leg, regulate qi and blood of the zang-fu organs by activating corresponding points and achieve health.

祛 病 健 身

Removes diseases and promotes health

通过长期的教学与临床实践证明，本功法锻炼既可扶助正气，又可祛除邪气，能够起到祛病健身的作用，长期习练本功法能调理三焦、疏肝、健脾，对虚证内脏下垂、高血压、肠胃病、便秘、内分泌失调以及免疫功能低下等病症有较好的防治作用。习练天柱摆动法还能防治颈椎、胸椎、腰椎增生病，脊椎小关节紊乱等退行性疾病，它能自我牵引脊柱，朝四个方向摆动脊柱，帮助纠正体形，强健体魄；习练三紧法可防治虚证内脏下垂、肠胃病、便秘、内分泌失调以及免疫功能低下等病症；习练三松法可以防治高血压、老慢支、焦虑症、抑郁症等疾病。

Education and clinical practice have proven that this exercise can supplement healthy qi, remove pathogenic qi, eliminate diseases and benefit health. Persistent exercise can regulate *Sanjiao*, soothe the liver, strengthen the spleen and prevent or treat visceroptosis, hypotension, gastrointestinal disorders, constipation, endocrine disorder and immunodeficiency. *Tian Zhu* swing exercise can prevent or treat degenerative cervical, thoracic, lumbar vertebral hyperplasia and spinal facet joint disorders. The three-relaxed method can prevent or treat hypertension, chronic bronchitis, anxiety and depression.

天 柱 导 引 功 ・ *Tian Zhu Dao Yin Gong*

The Meridian Charts

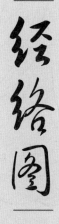

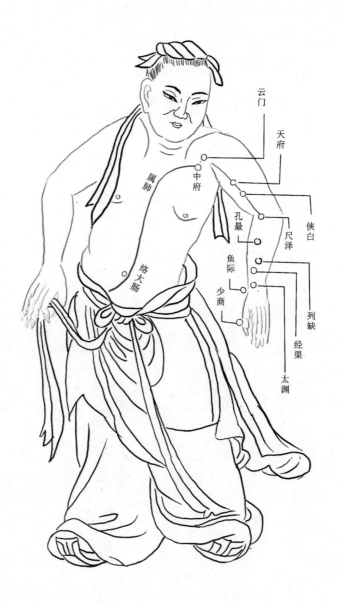

云门
天府
中府
属肺
侠白
孔最
尺泽
鱼际
经大肠
少商
列缺
经渠
太渊

手太阴肺经

Lung Meridian of Hand-Taiyin

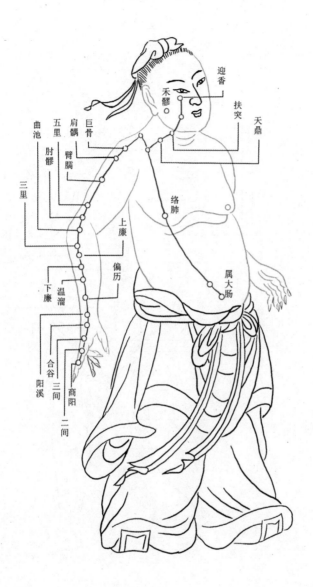

手阳明大肠经

Large Intestine Meridian of Hand-Yangming

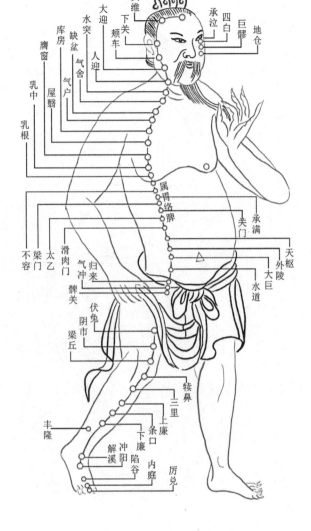

足阳明胃经

Stomach Meridian of Foot-Yangming

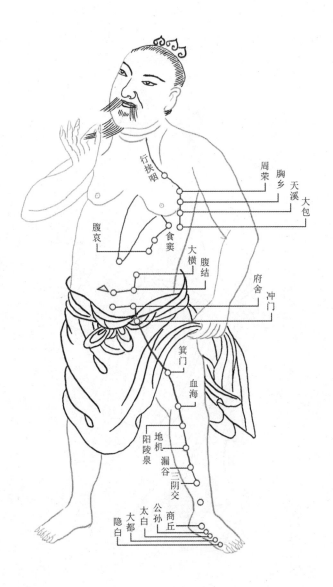

足太阴脾经

Spleen Meridian of Foot-Taiyin

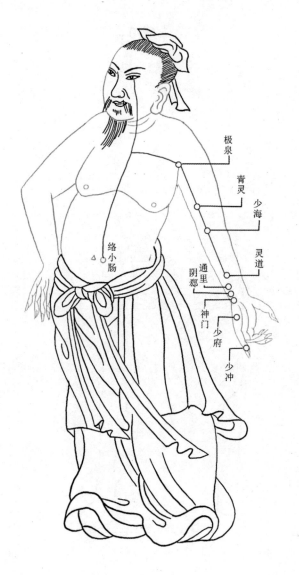

极泉

青灵

少海

灵道

通里

阴郄

神门

少府

少冲

络小肠

手少阴心经

Heart Meridian of Hand-Shaoyin

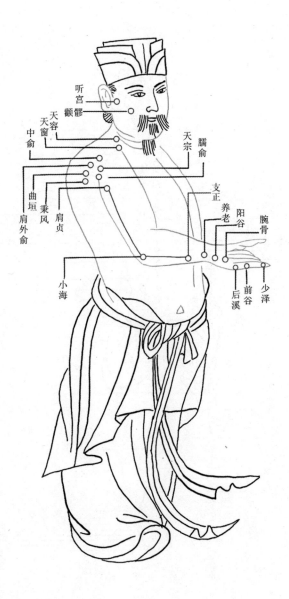

手太阳小肠经

Small Intestine Meridian of Hand-Taiyang

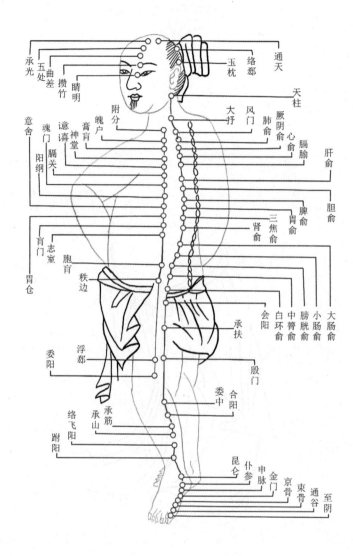

足太阳膀胱经

Bladder Meridian of Foot-Taiyang

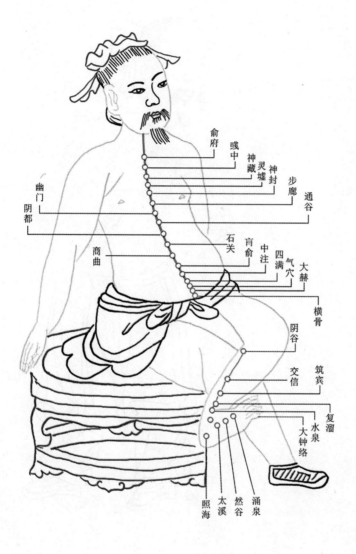

俞府
彧中
神藏
灵墟
神封
步廊
通谷
幽门
阴都
商曲
石关
肓俞
中注
气穴
四满
大赫
横骨
阴谷
交信
筑宾
复溜
水泉
大钟络
照海
然谷
太溪
涌泉

足少阴肾经

Kidney Meridian of Foot-Shaoyin

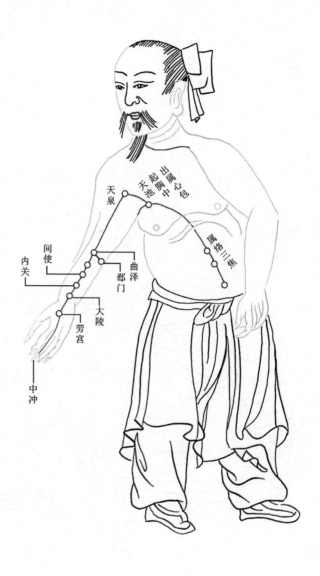

手厥阴心包经

Pericardium Meridian of Hand-Jueyin

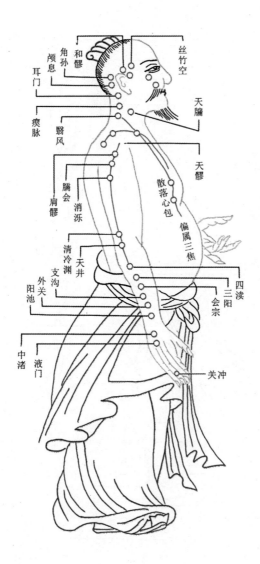

角孙　和髎　　　　　丝竹空
颅息
耳门　　　　　　　　　天牖
瘈脉
　　翳风
　　　　　　　　　天髎
臑会　　散落心包
肩髎　消泺
　　　　　　偏属三焦
清冷渊　天井
外关　支沟　　三阳　四渎
阳池　　　　　会宗
中渚　液门
　　　　　　关冲

手少阳三焦经

Triple Energizer Meridian of Hand-Shaoyang

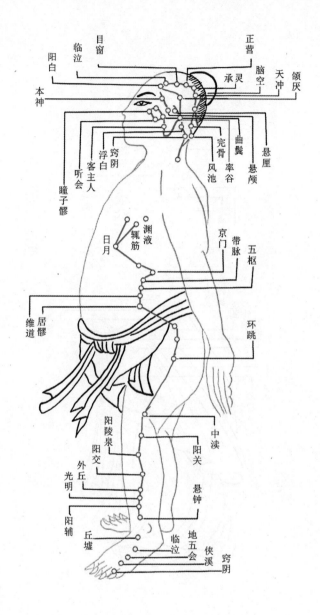

正营
脑空
天冲
颌厌
承灵
目窗
临泣
阳白
悬厘
曲鬓
率谷
悬颅
完骨
本神
风池
窍阴
浮白
客主人
听会
瞳子髎
渊液
辄筋
日月
京门
带脉
五枢
环跳
维道
居髎
阳陵泉
中渎
阳关
阳交
外丘
光明
悬钟
阳辅
丘墟
临泣
地五会
侠溪
窍阴

足少阳胆经

Gallbladder Meridian of Foot-Shaoyang

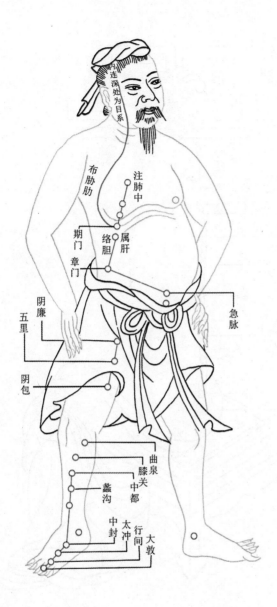

足厥阴肝经

Liver Meridian of Foot-Jueyin

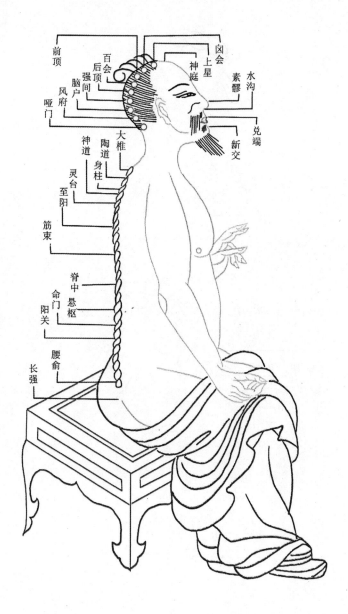

前顶
百会
后顶
强间
脑户
风府
哑门
囟会
上星
神庭
素髎
水沟
兑端
龈交
大椎
陶道
身柱
神道
灵台
至阳
筋束
脊中 悬枢
命门
阳关
腰俞
长强

督脉

Governor Vessel (Du)

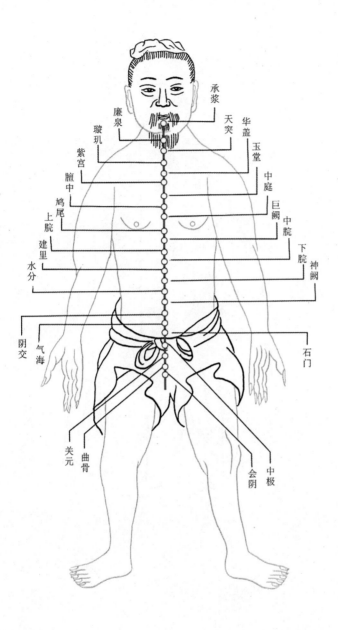

任脉

Conception Vessel (Ren)

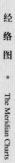
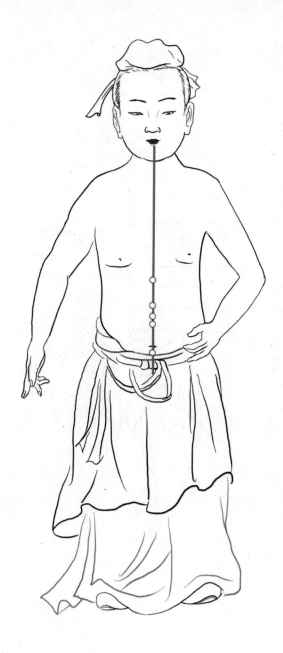

冲脉

Thoroughfare Vessel (Chong)

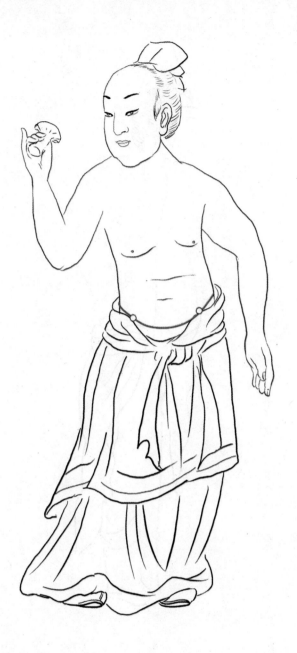

带脉

Belt Vessel (Dai)

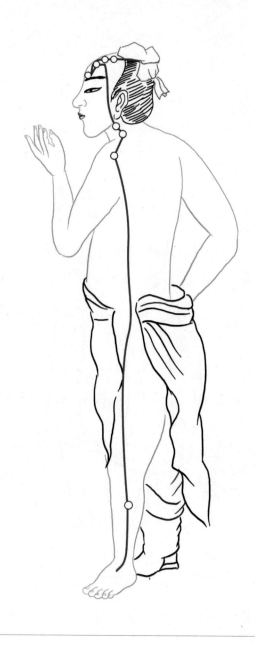

阳维脉

Yang Link Vessel (Yang Wei)

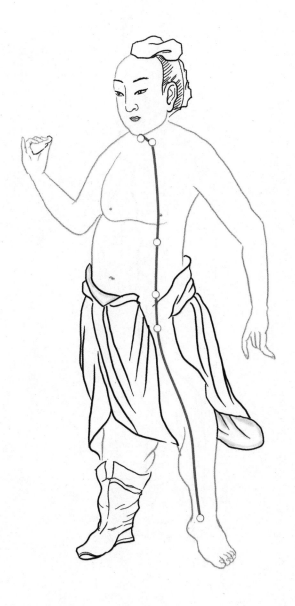

阴维脉

Yin Link Vessel (Yin Wei)

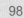
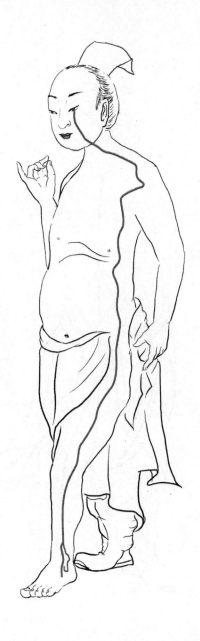

阳蹻脉

Yang Heel Vessel (Yang Qiao)

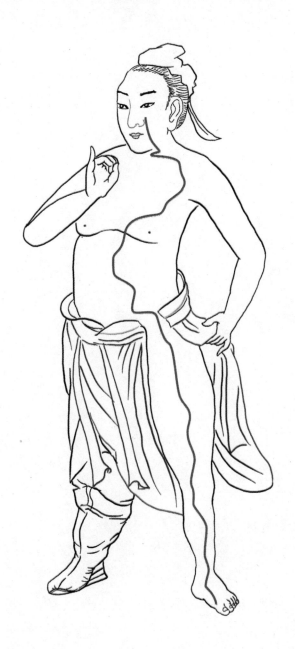

阴蹻脉

Yin Heel Vessel (Yin Qiao)